HAIR LOSS
Treatment

A 100% Natural Solution for Hair Growth and Hair Thinning Prevention Due to Alopecia in Men and Women

Alex G.O.

CONTENTS

UNDERSTANDING ALOPECIA: THE GLOBAL IMPACT OF HAIR LOSS

Alopecia is the medical term for hair loss, a condition that affects millions of people worldwide. While often associated with men, alopecia is also a significant concern for women. This widespread issue stems from a variety of causes and has implications that extend beyond the physical, often deeply affecting self-esteem and confidence. For younger individuals, in particular, hair loss can lead to distress, depression, and even social isolation.

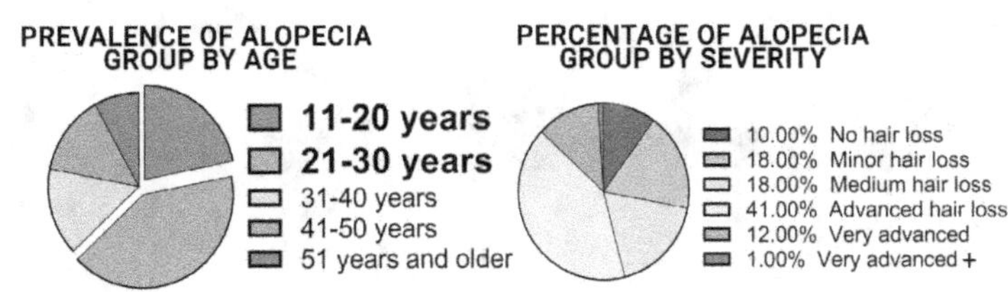

This book focuses on the most well-known form of alopecia: androgenetic alopecia, which accounts for 95% of hair loss cases in men and approximately 60% in women. This condition is linked to hormonal and genetic factors. Among men, androgenetic alopecia typically begins around the age of 20 and progresses over time. Research shows that approximately 40% of men aged 18 to 39 experience this condition, with the prevalence increasing to an astounding 95% among men over 70.

In women, androgenetic alopecia is generally less noticeable and manifests more diffusely, which can make early diagnosis challenging. Nonetheless, around 12% of women over 70 experience visible hair loss, and studies estimate that up to 50% of women will face some form of alopecia during their lifetime.

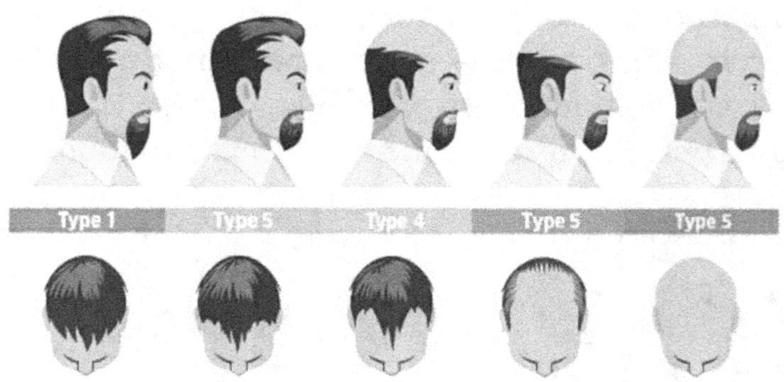

As the most common type of hair loss globally, alopecia carries not just physical consequences but emotional and psychological ones as well. Hair plays a crucial role in personal identity and self-image. In many cultures, it is strongly associated with beauty and attractiveness, both to oneself and to others. These societal pressures can make hair loss a source of significant emotional distress.

The good news is that there are natural and effective solutions to prevent and treat alopecia. These methods can not only help you restore your hair but also allow you to regain your confidence.

In this book, I will introduce you to natural approaches that can transform your hair health safely and effectively. Whether you're a man or a woman, whether you're just beginning to notice hair loss or have been dealing with it for some time, the following chapters will equip you with the knowledge and tools needed to regain control over your hair health completely naturally.

THE SCIENCE OF HAIR LOSS: GENETICS, HORMONES, AND MORE

Hair loss is something we all face at some point in our lives, but understanding why it happens is key to addressing the issue effectively. In this chapter, I want to share with you the scientific foundations behind alopecia and hair loss so that you can better understand how it affects your body and, more importantly, how you can tackle it naturally.

Remember: the goal isn't just to find a quick fix. What's truly important is understanding the problem and building a solid "why" that allows you to become fully aware of what you need to do to make the change you desire. Your desire to change must be stronger than your desire to stay where you are.

First, it's essential to talk about genetics, as it plays a major role in hair loss. Androgenetic alopecia, or common baldness, is the most common type of hair loss in both men and women. If you have a family history of hair loss, it's likely that you'll inherit this predisposition. This is simply the genetic information passed down through generations, which can cause hair follicles to shrink over time, leading to thinner, less dense hair.

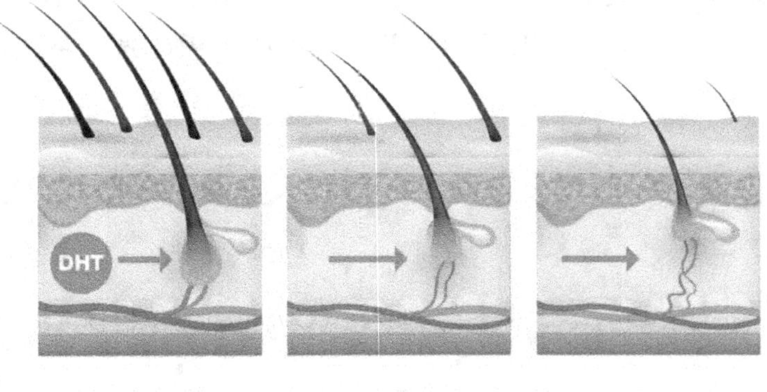

But genetics isn't the only factor at play. Hormones also have a significant impact, particularly in both male and female hair loss. In men, dihydrotestosterone (DHT), a hormone derived from testosterone, is the main culprit behind the miniaturization of hair follicles. In women, hormonal imbalances related to the menstrual cycle, pregnancy, or menopause can trigger hair loss. Hormonal fluctuations affect the natural growth cycle of hair, causing it to weaken and fall out.

In the following chapters, we'll explore how you can use both natural techniques and products to slow down and even reverse hair loss, targeting the root cause based on the principles I've just explained.

I'll provide straightforward, practical advice so you don't have to read through a 300-page book to address a problem that can be solved with relatively simple remedies, as long as you maintain the right solutions and adapt simple routines to your daily life.

THE ROLE OF LIFESTYLE AND STRESS IN HAIR HEALTH

In addition to genetics and hormones, factors such as stress, diet, hair care, and even the environment play a crucial role in hair health. These factors can disrupt the natural balance of your scalp, accelerating hair loss or causing excessive thinning.

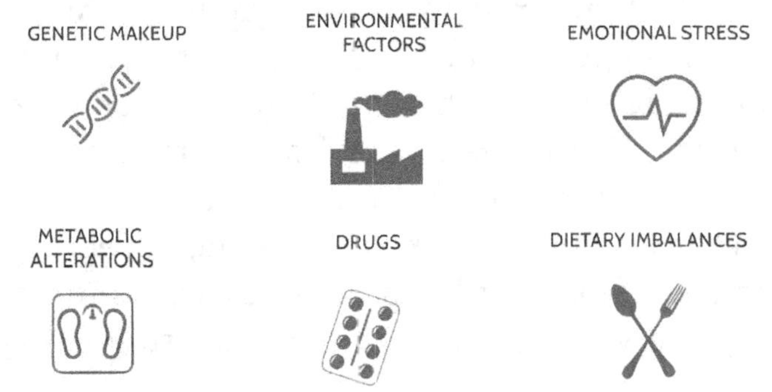

Understanding these factors is the first step in taking control of your hair health, allowing you to identify which elements are negatively affecting you and where you have full control to make changes.

Stress is one of the most powerful factors influencing hair loss. When you experience high levels of stress, your body produces more cortisol, a hormone that, in excess, can cause hair follicles to enter an early resting phase, known as telogen effluvium. Recent studies show that up to 30% of people who undergo a traumatic event or suffer from chronic stress experience significant hair loss. This type of hair loss is often reversible, but without proper stress management, it becomes a cycle that is difficult to break.

Nutrition is also essential; if you are not getting the necessary nutrients (such as vitamins, minerals, and proteins) your hair will suffer the consequences. Nutrients like iron, B vitamins (such as biotin), and zinc are vital for strengthening hair follicles and promoting healthy growth. A diet rich in fresh, natural foods, such as fruits, vegetables, lean proteins, and healthy fats, can be key to improving your hair's health. Current research suggests that vitamin D and iron deficiencies are linked to a higher risk of alopecia, especially in women. If your diet lacks these essential nutrients, your hair will be the first to show it, losing strength and thickness.

Of course, lifestyle habits like smoking or excessive alcohol consumption also affect blood circulation to the scalp, weakening hair follicles and accelerating hair loss.

In addition to lifestyle, environmental factors such as pollution and physical damage also affect hair health. Exposure to pollutants, especially in urban environments, damages the hair cuticle, making it more prone to dryness and breakage. A recent study in Asia showed that air pollution can accelerate hair damage by up to 20% compared to less polluted environments.

This is compounded by harsh chemicals and the excessive use of heat tools like blow dryers and straighteners. Frequent combing or products containing sulfates and parabens can wear down the hair cuticle, weakening it and promoting hair loss.

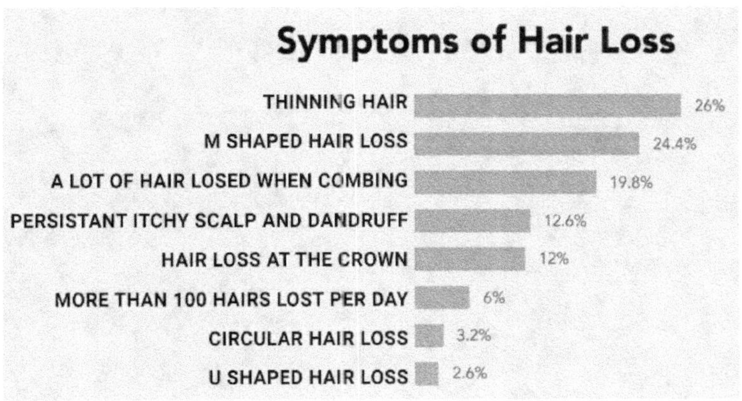

Consider these factors as pieces of a puzzle. Making adjustments to how you manage stress, improving your diet, and limiting the use of harsh products can protect and strengthen your hair. Small changes, such as practicing relaxation techniques, maintaining a balanced diet, and avoiding damaging habits, can be transformative.

Now that you're aware of these factors, I encourage you to consider these adjustments to give your body (and, of course, your hair) a much-needed break.

And don't worry, in a couple of chapters, we'll clearly define which nutrients you should be taking, from what food sources, and other key guidelines to ensure your scalp gets the essential nutrients it needs to stay strong, healthy, and stimulate your hair follicles.

TRADITIONAL TREATMENTS: PROS, CONS, AND ALTERNATIVES

When it comes to alopecia, several conventional treatments are widely used, such as minoxidil, finasteride, dutasteride, and advanced options like hair transplants. In this chapter, I want to explain how these treatments work, their disadvantages, limitations, and how they compare to natural alternatives.

Minoxidil is a topical medication, though it is now also available in oral form, that helps stimulate hair growth and increase hair thickness. It is applied directly to the scalp, and studies show that around 40-60% of users experience some degree of improvement after 3 to 6 months of use. However, the effects are temporary: once discontinued, the hair returns to its initial state. Common side effects include itching, dryness, or scalp irritation.

On the other hand, finasteride and dutasteride are oral pills that work by reducing the conversion of testosterone into DHT, the hormone responsible for hair loss in androgenetic alopecia. Both inhibit the enzyme 5-alpha reductase, but finasteride only blocks type II of this enzyme, while dutasteride inhibits both type I and type II. Studies indicate that around 66% of men see a reduction in hair loss with finasteride, but it is less effective in women and can cause side effects like reduced libido, erectile dysfunction, and, in rare cases, depression. As for dutasteride, the effects are more pronounced, both positively on hair growth and negatively in terms of side effects.

Lastly, hair transplants are often considered by many as a definitive solution to alopecia. However, it's important to note that it is an invasive treatment that doesn't address the underlying cause of hair loss. In this surgical procedure, hair follicles are extracted from a donor area (usually the back of the head) and transplanted to areas affected by alopecia. It is seen as an effective and long-term solution for those seeking a direct fix for hair loss. However, results are not immediate. Patients typically start to see visible results between 6 to 12 months post-surgery, as transplanted follicles need time to adapt to their new environment and begin to grow naturally.

Initially, the transplanted hairs go through a temporary shedding phase (known as "shock loss"), followed by a slow growth period. Within the first three months, the follicles settle in and start producing new hair, and it's usually around six months that significant improvements in hair density and thickness become noticeable.

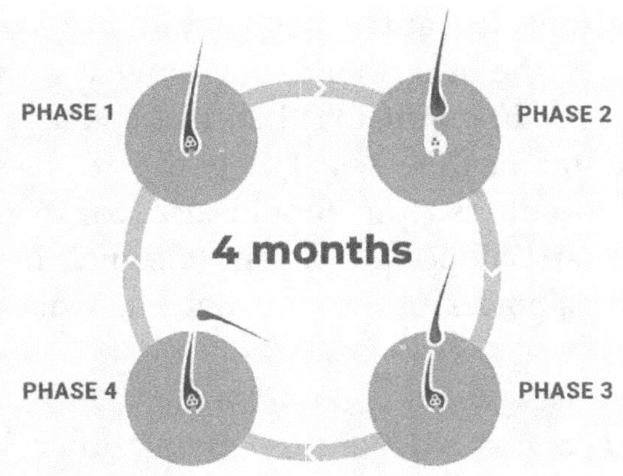

While hair transplants can offer permanent results in the treated areas, the underlying cause of androgenetic alopecia remains. This means that the issue of hair loss, driven by DHT (dihydrotestosterone), is not resolved with a transplant. Therefore, the transplant only improves hair density in the areas where the follicles are placed, but it does not stop hair loss in other parts of the scalp.

Knowing this, I think anyone reading these lines would agree that taking a pill for life isn't appealing when there are natural alternatives that offer the same benefits without the drawbacks, right?

The pharmaceutical industry thrives on selling processed compounds derived from plants, roots, trees, and fruits. It's simple: the pharmaceutical industry doesn't want you to know where they extract their ingredients for heavily processed formulations, because they would lose a lot of money. On the other hand, you don't want to take harmful products for life that affect your physical and mental health. Yes, I'm going to reveal the natural products you should use to solve your androgenetic alopecia problem (cheaper, healthier, and just as powerful for your hair) as what they're selling.

And that's not to mention many other healing solutions that don't come from Mother Nature but still promote hair growth. These I'll explain in detail next.

THE POWER OF NATURE: NATURAL TREATMENTS TO COMBAT ALOPECIA

Skin Absorption

In the search for solutions to combat alopecia, essential oils are among the most valuable resources at our disposal. These oils, extracted from plants, have properties that stimulate hair growth and improve scalp health in a safe and effective way. In this section, I'll explain how they work and how you can incorporate them into your hair care routine.

Essential oils like rosemary, lavender, peppermint, and tea tree oil have the ability to penetrate the scalp due to their small molecular structure, allowing them to be absorbed by the skin and act directly on the hair follicles. For example, rosemary oil has been the subject of recent studies comparing it to minoxidil in its ability to improve hair density. A study published in the Journal of Dermatology showed that rosemary was just as effective as minoxidil in stimulating hair growth in patients with androgenetic alopecia, but without the side effects of minoxidil.

Lavender oil is ideal for those with sensitive or inflamed scalps. With its relaxing and anti-inflammatory properties, a study in the Journal of Ethnopharmacology showed that its application in animals promoted significant hair growth and improved scalp health due to its calming effects. Peppermint oil, on the other hand, is known for its ability to improve blood circulation in the scalp. A study published in Toxicological Research found that peppermint oil stimulated hair growth in mice by increasing the flow of nutrients and oxygen to the hair follicles, contributing to stronger, healthier hair.

Tea tree oil is particularly useful for cases of dandruff or scalp infections because it is both antimicrobial and antifungal. These indirect benefits help keep the scalp healthy, a key factor in reducing hair loss. Other oils, such as pumpkin seed oil, have been shown to partially block the action of dihydrotestosterone (DHT), a hormone associated with androgenetic alopecia.

Thyme oil and cedarwood oil have also shown positive effects in cases of alopecia areata. A study in Archives of Dermatology found that this combination of essential oils helped reverse hair loss in people with this condition due to their stimulating and antimicrobial effects.

Finally, castor oil, rich in ricinoleic acid (an anti-inflammatory and antimicrobial fatty acid) helps keep the scalp healthy. Additionally, castor oil improves blood circulation and strengthens the hair, promoting thicker, more robust hair growth.

To harness these benefits, I suggest mixing a few drops of these essential oils with a carrier oil like coconut or jojoba oil and massaging it into your scalp. This massage not only facilitates the absorption of the nutrients but also improves circulation in the area and helps reduce stress, which, as we know, also plays a role in hair loss.

Incorporating these oils into your routine is simple and affordable, and unlike many conventional treatments, they come with no side effects unless you have an allergy, which is rare, less than 1% of people experience any allergic reactions.

Essential Foods and Nutrients

A balanced diet is crucial for keeping your hair healthy and strong, as the nutrients we obtain from food provide the necessary building blocks for hair growth and strength. Here's a guide to foods rich in essential nutrients like iron, protein, omega-3s, and antioxidants, which play a key role in preventing hair loss and fortifying your hair.

Iron is essential for oxygen transport in the blood and is crucial for hair growth, as it helps deliver sufficient oxygen and nutrients to the hair follicles. Foods rich in iron include spinach, legumes, red meat, and liver. Including these in your diet is particularly important if you tend to have low iron levels, which is common in people with alopecia. Studies have shown that iron deficiency is linked to an increased likelihood of hair loss.

Hair is primarily made up of keratin, a structural protein, so consuming enough protein is key to its health. I recommend adding eggs, chicken, fish, and legumes to your diet as excellent sources of protein. These help maintain the structure of your hair and prevent it from breaking or getting damaged. A lack of protein can cause your hair to weaken and, over time, lead to increased shedding.

Omega-3 fatty acids are anti-inflammatory and essential for the scalp, helping keep it hydrated and reducing dryness that may contribute to hair loss. You can find omega-3s in foods like salmon, walnuts, flaxseeds, and chia seeds. Recent studies highlight that a diet rich in omega-3s helps reduce hair loss by strengthening hair follicles and improving circulation to the scalp.

Antioxidants protect the hair from free radicals, which can damage the follicles and hinder hair growth. Fruits and vegetables like strawberries, oranges, carrots, and spinach are excellent sources of antioxidants such as vitamins C and E. Adding these foods to your diet helps strengthen your hair from the root, providing protection against environmental damage and oxidative stress.

And be mindful: these changes won't just improve the health of your hair; they are not about following a strict diet, but about making gradual and sustainable additions that will not only strengthen your hair but also boost your overall energy, health, and mood. You don't have to do everything at once, start small adapting what works for you. Taking care of your body is an act of self-love. You're taking steps toward a healthier, more balanced life, where every small effort counts in improving your overall well-being.

I hope this extra resource and this book, along with your desire to improve your hair health, leads you to discover how to also develop, nurture, and enhance many other areas of your life.

Additional Supplements

As a natural complement taken orally, I want to highlight and give special attention to saw palmetto (Serenoa repens). Saw palmetto is an extract from the fruit of the American dwarf palm, and it has shown effectiveness in combating androgenetic alopecia by inhibiting the enzyme 5-alpha reductase, which converts testosterone into DHT (dihydrotestosterone), the hormone responsible for hair loss. By reducing DHT levels, saw palmetto helps prevent damage to hair follicles, stopping hair loss and promoting healthier hair growth.

Saw palmetto is one of the most studied supplements for androgenetic alopecia, with numerous studies backing its effectiveness. One study published in The Journal of Alternative and Complementary Medicine demonstrated that saw palmetto is just as effective as finasteride in halting hair loss, but without the typical side effects associated with this medication.

It's important to note that the side effects linked to saw palmetto are generally mild and primarily gastrointestinal, occurring in just about 2% of the population. There may also be interactions with certain medications, such as blood thinners or exogenous hormone treatments. As always, this information should not replace medical advice, so it's essential to consult a healthcare professional before starting any supplement regimen.

The recommended daily dose ranges between 160 and 320 mg, and saw palmetto is commonly available in capsule or liquid extract form. This natural treatment offers an attractive option because it addresses the hormonal causes of hair loss without the high incidence or severity of side effects seen with conventional medications. While results may take a few months to appear, saw palmetto is a safe and effective alternative for improving scalp health.

Physical Effects

If you're looking for a non-invasive, science-backed approach to stimulate hair growth, red LED light therapy could be an interesting option. Known as low-level light therapy (LLLT), this treatment uses specific wavelengths of red light to penetrate the scalp and improve the health of hair follicles.

Red LED light works by stimulating blood circulation in the scalp, allowing more oxygen and nutrients to reach the follicles. This increase in blood flow helps revitalize dormant follicles and strengthen existing hair. Additionally, LLLT promotes the production of cellular energy (ATP) in the hair follicle cells, encouraging a healthier hair cycle.

Studies have shown promising results. For instance, research published in the American Journal of Clinical Dermatology found that regular use of red light devices significantly improved hair density in patients with androgenetic alopecia. Another study in the Journal of Cosmetic and Laser Therapy showed that participants experienced thicker hair and increased hair count after 26 weeks of LLLT treatment. (Studies have shown that both LED and laser treatments can be effective)

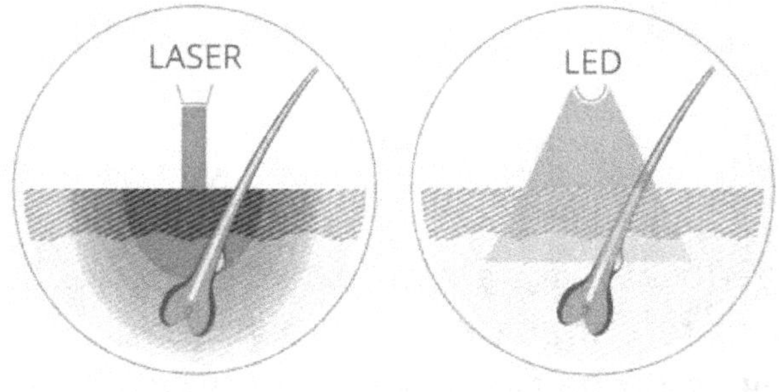

The best part of this approach is its safety. Unlike some medications, LLLT has no known side effects and can be easily used at home with approved devices. As with any treatment (including hair transplants), consistency is key. Results typically begin to show after 3 to 6 months of regular use, so establishing a routine is essential.

If you decide to try red LED light therapy, make sure to consult with a specialist to select the right device and tailor a plan that meets your needs.

Dermaroller

The dermaroller has gained popularity as a non-invasive tool for treating hair loss, especially in cases of androgenetic alopecia. This device, covered with tiny needles, stimulates the scalp through a process called microneedling, which creates small incisions in the skin to activate cellular regeneration, promote collagen production (Collagen Induction Therapy, CIT), increase blood flow, and enhance the absorption of topical treatments such as essential oils.

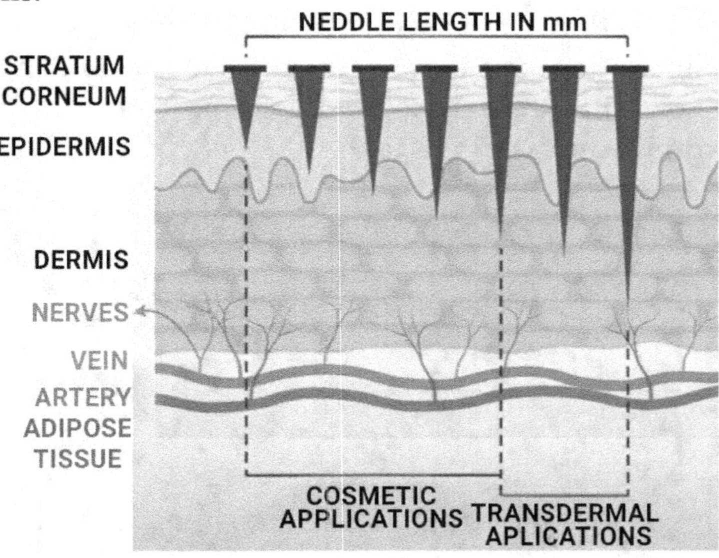

The size of the needles is crucial for the device's effectiveness and safety. Typically, needle sizes between 0.25 mm and 1.5 mm are recommended for the scalp. Smaller needles (0.25 mm) are ideal for beginners or those with sensitive skin, as well as for enhancing the absorption of topical products, while larger needles (1.0–1.5 mm) are more effective at stimulating the hair follicles. My advice is to start with smaller needles (0.25–0.5 mm) and gradually progress to 1mm.

There are also devices such as the dermastamp and dermapen, which, although slightly more expensive, eliminate the margin of error when applying the correct angle (in the case of the dermastamp) or ensuring the proper depth of skin penetration (in the case of the dermapen). By eliminating any human error, scientific evidence shows that 0.5 mm needles are the most effective for stimulating hair growth.

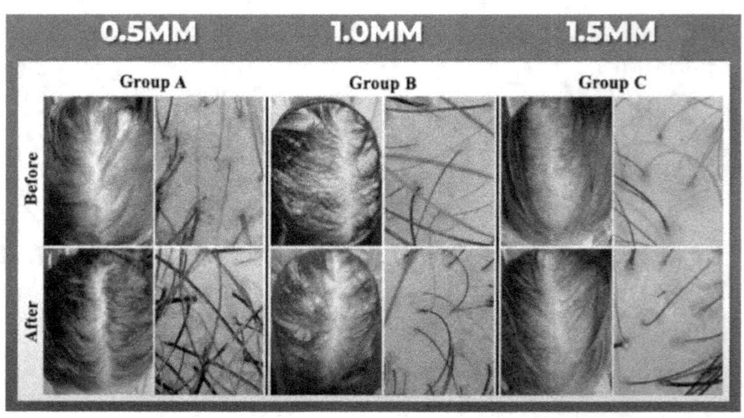

Medhat W. Rezk AF. Assesing the efficacy

of automated microneedling monotherapy for androgenetic alopecia. A comparison of 3 different depths.

For optimal results, it's important to use the dermaroller 1 to 2 times per week, allowing your scalp to recover between sessions. During use, move the device in multiple directions (vertically, horizontally, and diagonally) to cover the entire affected area, making 6 to 10 passes per section. Be sure to avoid applying excessive pressure to prevent damage to the skin.

As I mentioned earlier, the dermaroller not only improves circulation but also boosts the effectiveness of topical treatments. A study published in the International Journal of Trichology found that combining the dermaroller with minoxidil resulted in a doubling of hair density compared to using the medication alone. Therefore, if essential oils have similar effectiveness to minoxidil, they will also have a significantly enhanced effect when used with the dermaroller.

Always remember to disinfect the device before and after each use to prevent infections. You can simply immerse the needle head in boiling water or spray it with alcohol. And, like with any treatment, be sure to consult with a professional before adding it to your routine. The dermaroller can be a powerful ally if used consistently and with care.

SELF-CARE ROUTINES AND PRACTICES FOR HEALTHY HAIR

Techniques to Reduce Stress

Taking care of your hair goes far beyond the products we apply. The connection between the body and mind plays a crucial role in hair health, and managing cortisol levels the stress hormone can be key to preventing hair loss. Daily life, with its demands and challenges, increases cortisol production in our bodies, which, over time, can harm not only hair growth but also hair strength. I want to share some practices that can help reduce stress and improve the well-being of both your hair and overall health.

Meditation, while simple, is a powerful tool for calming the mind and reducing cortisol levels. Spending just a few minutes each day focusing on deep breathing and being present in the moment can have a profound effect on your hair health. Recent studies have shown that daily meditation can reduce cortisol levels by up to 20%. If you're new to meditation, mobile apps or online tutorials are a great place to start.

Exercise, in addition to its physical benefits, is also an excellent stress regulator. When you exercise, the body releases endorphins, known as the "happy hormones," which counteract the effects of cortisol. Activities like yoga, outdoor walks, or swimming, when practiced regularly, are effective in reducing stress and improving blood circulation, which, in turn, benefits the scalp.

Finally, getting enough sleep is another crucial habit. Lack of sleep increases cortisol levels, and the quality of sleep directly impacts hair health. Try to maintain a regular sleep routine and create a restful environment, as this contributes to stronger hair.

These simple but effective practices can be the first step toward long-term hair health. Incorporating them into your daily routine will not only take care of your hair but also improve your general well-being.

Scalp Massage Exercises

Sometimes, the most effective solutions for hair loss are also the simplest. Scalp massage is an ancient practice that is not only soothing but also a powerful tool to stimulate hair growth. By massaging the scalp, you improve blood circulation to the follicles, creating an optimal environment for them to stay active and healthy. Additionally, massage can enhance the absorption of topical treatments such as essential oils or serums, making it the perfect time to apply these products.

Scientific studies support this practice. One study published in Eplasty showed that massaging the scalp daily for four minutes over a 24-week period helped increase hair density in participants.

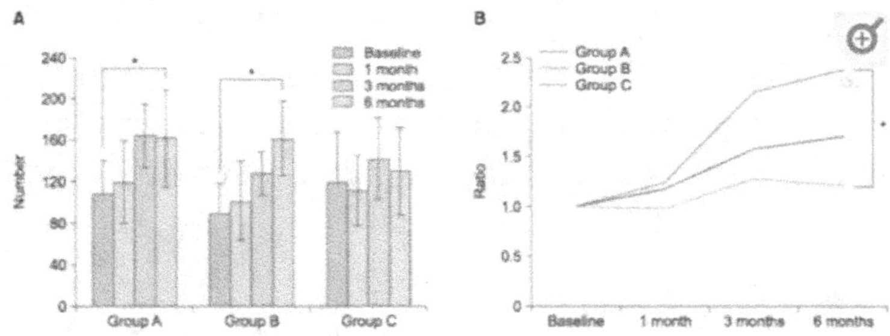

Hair count. (A) An increase in hair count for 6 months was 52.6 in group A ($^*p<0.05$), 71.5 in group B ($^*p<0.05$), and 9.6 in group C. (B) The ratio of changes in hair count between group B (n=2.38) and group C (n=1.21) only at 6 months showed a statistically significant difference ($^*p<0.05$).

If you want to incorporate this technique into your routine, here are several effective methods:

N°1 Circular Finger Technique: Use the pads of your fingers to make gentle circular motions all over your scalp. Start from the hairline and move towards the crown, applying moderate pressure.

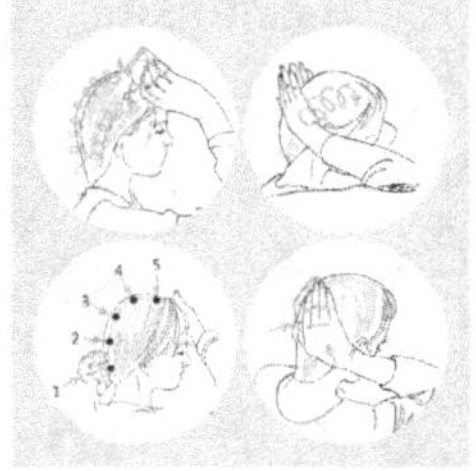

N°2 Pressure and Relaxation Method: Place the palms of your hands on both sides of your head and apply light pressure for a second before releasing. Repeat this motion in different areas.

Spending just a few minutes each day on this practice is easy, relaxing, and highly beneficial. Scalp massage not only helps care for your hair but is also an excellent way to reduce stress, another enemy of hair health. With this new addition of scalp massage, you'll benefit from increased absorption of essential oils, enhanced follicle stimulation, and reduced stress a natural 3-in-1 that will help in your journey toward stronger hair.

I'm attaching an explanatory video about different types of massages. I recommend:

#1: After applying oils.
#3: When drying your hair.
#12: As a daily routine.

Scalp massage is a natural technique designed to alleviate tension in the head while encouraging vasodilation and improving blood circulation to the scalp and hair follicles. This process mirrors the mechanisms of treatments such as minoxidil, which functions as a vasodilator to enhance blood flow; PRP (Platelet-Rich Plasma), which replenishes blood in targeted areas; and Botox injections, which relax scalp muscles to facilitate oxygen and nutrient delivery. Despite their different methods, these approaches share the same objective: boosting local circulation to foster a healthier scalp and stimulate optimal hair growth.

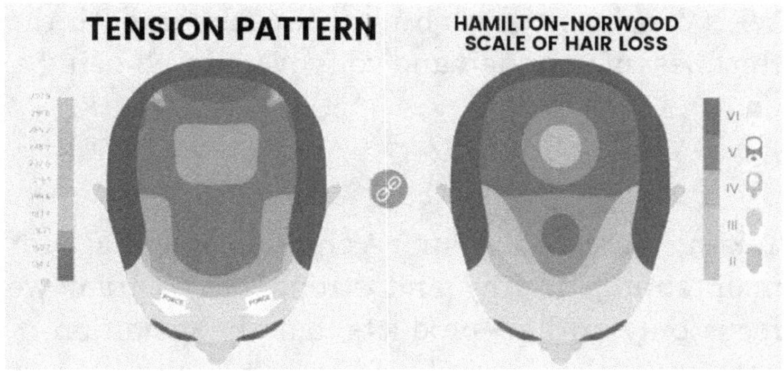

Research indicates that daily scalp massages lasting at least 4 minutes can significantly enhance hair thickness and improve scalp elasticity, while also reducing fibrosis. For even greater benefits, longer sessions of 5 to 10 minutes per day are recommended, as they further stimulate blood flow, reduce tension, and enhance the health of hair follicles.

One of the greatest advantages of scalp massage is that its effects improve with consistent practice. Unlike other treatments, it doesn't have a fixed efficacy limit based on usage time. With regular, extended sessions, you increase the likelihood of achieving optimal results.

My recommendation? Incorporate two daily sessions, one in the morning and another in the evening, each lasting 4–5 minutes for the best outcomes.

With consistency, you'll notice results in both the thickness of your hair and your overall well-being.

Daily Scalp Care

Taking care of your scalp is essential for maintaining healthy and strong hair. Often, we focus only on hair products, but the condition of your scalp plays a vital role in hair health. If your scalp isn't clean, hydrated, and free from irritants, hair follicles can't function properly. Here are some tips to help you take care of your scalp every day.

First, it's important to cleanse your scalp regularly, but without overdoing it. Just like the rest of your skin, your scalp needs to be cleaned to prevent the buildup of sebum, dead skin cells, and product residues. However, washing your hair too often can have the opposite effect. The more you wash your hair, the more sebum your scalp will produce in response to the loss of natural oils. The trick is to find balance: it's not necessary to wash your hair every day, especially if you have a sensitive scalp. For most people, washing hair 2 to 3 times a week is sufficient.

Choosing the right shampoo is crucial. Today, there are mobile apps that allow you to scan cosmetic products and check whether they contain harmful ingredients. These apps can help you choose products free of sulfates and parabens, which are known to be harsh on both the scalp and hair as they can cause dryness and irritation. By opting for natural products without aggressive chemicals, you'll help maintain the balance of your scalp's skin, preventing overproduction of sebum.

Hydration is also key. If your scalp is dry, it can cause itching and inflammation, which negatively affects hair health. Use products that won't overload your hair but will provide essential nutrients, such as natural oils like jojoba or coconut oil, which keep the skin hydrated without clogging the pores.

Remember, gentleness matters. Avoid scrubbing your scalp too aggressively when washing your hair; instead, as we've seen, perform a gentle scalp massage with the pads of your fingers. It's not just about what you do but also about how you do it.

Incorporating these practices into your daily routine will help maintain a healthy scalp, and ultimately, strong, beautiful hair.

SUCCESS STORIES: REAL CASES OF HAIR RESTORATION

In this section, I'd like to share some case studies that highlight the tangible results achieved through natural hair loss treatments. Through "before" and "after" images, you'll see how different individuals have experienced remarkable improvements in their hair health. (4-6 months of evolution).

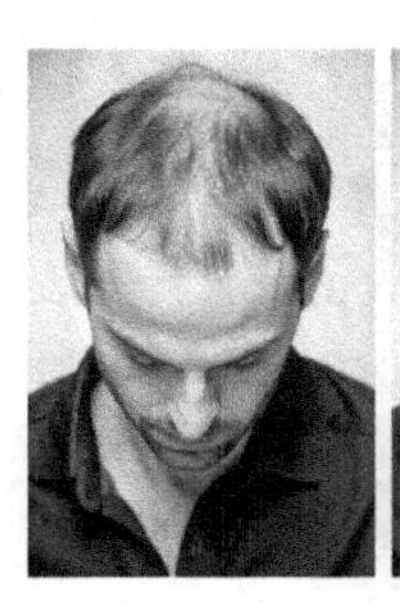
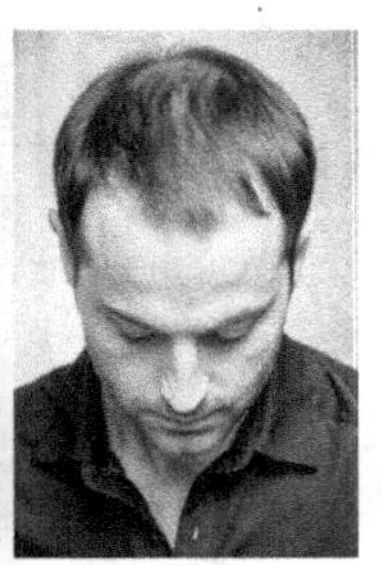
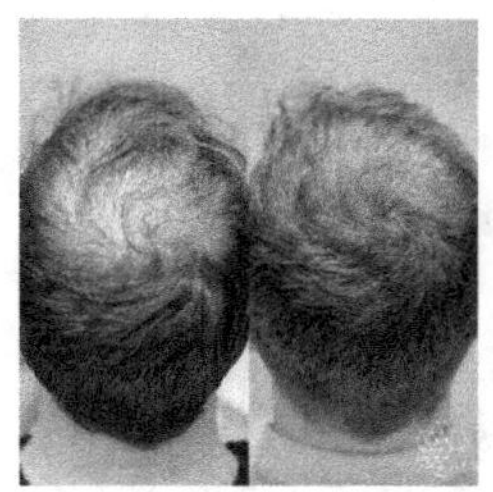
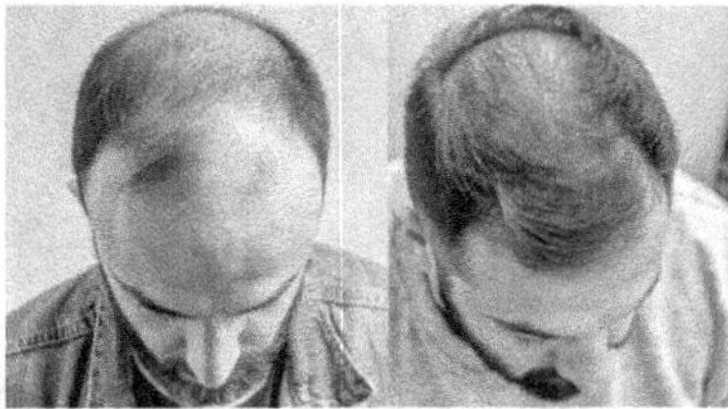

These stories these stories through photographs and hundred of studies not only demonstrate the positive impact of these treatments but also reflect the dedication and consistency required to achieve effective results. Each testimonial serves as a reminder that, with the right approach, patience, and commitment, it's possible to regain confidence and improve your hair's health. These treatments have transformed lives and could do the same for you.

Testimonials

"At first, it seemed like there were too many steps, and it was a bit overwhelming to manage. But once I started incorporating the treatments, I realized it was much simpler than I thought. Now, I've easily made them a part of my daily routine, and the results are clear."

"I'm really impressed with the scientifically-backed treatments in this book. Just using one of them already brought noticeable changes, and when you combine several, you benefit from the results of dozens of studies. It's amazing how something so simple can be so effective!"

"In just three months, I saw incredible changes in my hair. This book made my life so much easier. It's short but clear, with easy-to-follow guidelines, and the additional resources helped me take action. The progress has been much greater than I expected."

LONG-TERM MAINTENANCE GUIDE FOR HEALTHY HAIR

The journey to strong, healthy hair doesn't end once you start seeing results. In fact, it marks the beginning of a process that requires patience, consistency, and ongoing attention. Maintaining healthy hair in the long term is about caring for yourself from the inside out and adopting daily habits that help keep everything in balance.

Adopting a new lifestyle should not be seen as an obligation but as a conscious decision to achieve the life you desire. When you act with purpose, the effort fades away, as intention transforms the way you perceive and live your daily life.

Key Practices for Healthy Hair

- **Nutritional Support:** Incorporate iron-rich foods, proteins, B vitamins, omega-3s, and antioxidants into your diet to nourish your hair from within.
- **Supplements:** Consider supplements like saw palmetto, after consulting a professional.

- <u>Dermaroller Use:</u> Apply a dermaroller correctly to enhance cellular regeneration and the absorption of topical products.

- <u>Essential Oils:</u> Use rosemary, lavender, peppermint, or pumpkin seed oils to promote scalp health and stimulate hair growth.

- <u>Scalp Massage:</u> Make daily scalp massages part of your routine during shampooing or oil application to boost circulation and encourage growth.

- <u>Stress Management:</u> Practice relaxation techniques such as meditation, yoga, or exercise to reduce stress and ensure restful sleep.

- <u>Gentle Hair Care:</u> Avoid harsh treatments and opt for sulfate-free cosmetic products to maintain a clean, undamaged scalp.

- <u>Red Light Therapy:</u> Consider using red LED light to stimulate blood circulation and cellular regeneration in the scalp.

I've prepared a printable version of this so you can keep it handy in case you need it.

Above all, the most crucial takeaway is this: Maintaining strong, healthy hair requires a consistent, balanced routine. The regimen isn't demanding the true challenge lies in fostering the awareness and discipline to implement and sustain these habits over time.

To help you stay on track, I'm giving you this extra: a planner to manage your actions and progress throughout your journey.

A Cost-Effective Solution Compared to Hair Transplants

In the United States, individuals undergoing hair transplants spend an average of $4,000 to $20,000 USD, depending on their initial condition and the degree of hair loss. It's worth noting that these costs typically cover only the surgical procedure and exclude additional expenses such as medications, pre-op consultations, follow-ups, or post-op treatments. Furthermore, patients must continue taking medications to prevent future androgenic hair loss.

With these natural remedies and new habits, you will face:

- <u>Similar</u> (a little bit higher) maintenance responsibilities to those who undergo transplants.

- <u>Minimal</u> or no side effects, with an allergy or incompatibility rate of less than 2%.

- <u>Faster results:</u> Natural methods can deliver visible improvements in 3-6 months, versus 6-12 months with a transplant.

- <u>Significantly lower costs:</u> The total expense is limited to this book and the products you choose, with a combined cost of under $100.

This journey isn't just about improving your hair; it's about embracing a holistic approach to self-care and enhancing every aspect of your life. There's always a solution waiting to be discovered. Keep exploring, experimenting, and, most importantly, enjoy the process because the best results always begin with you.

BIBLIOGRAPHIC REFERENCES

- Adil A, Godwin M. The effectiveness of treatments for androgenetic alopecia: A systematic review and meta-analysis. J Am Acad Dermatol. 2017;77(1):136-141.e5. doi:10.1016/j.jaad.2017.02.054

- Owen K. Hair loss statistics (2024). Medihair. https://medihair.com/es/estadisticas-sobre-la-caida-del-cabello/. Publicado en 2024.

- Rossi A, Anzalone A, Fortuna MC, et al. Multi-therapies in androgenetic alopecia: review and clinical experiences. Dermatol Ther. 2016;29(6):424-432. doi:10.1111/dth.12390

- Olsen, E. A., Dunlap, F. E., Funicella, T., Koperski, J. A., Swinehart, J. M., Tschen, E. H., & Trancik, R. J. (2002). A randomized clinical trial of 5% topical minoxidil versus 2% topical minoxidil and placebo in the treatment of androgenetic alopecia in men. Journal of the American Academy of Dermatology, 47(3), 377–385. https://doi.org/10.1067/mjd.2002.123405

- Suchonwanit, P., Thammarucha, S., & Leerunyakul, K. (2019). Minoxidil and its use in hair disorders: A review. Drug Design, Development and

Therapy, 13, 2777–2786. https://doi.org/10.2147/DDDT.S214907

- Kaufman, K. D., & Olsen, E. A. (2008). Androgenetic alopecia. In Diseases of the Skin (pp. 925-945). Saunders.

- Irwig, M. S. (2012). Persistent sexual side effects of finasteride: Could they be permanent? Journal of Sexual Medicine, 9(11), 2927–2932. https://doi.org/10.1111/j.1743-6109.2012.02974.x

- Price, V. H. (1999). Treatment of hair loss. New England Journal of Medicine, 341(13), 964–973. https://doi.org/10.1056/NEJM199909233411307

- Bernstein, R. M., & Rassman, W. R. (2002). Follicular unit transplantation: 2002. Dermatologic Surgery, 28(9), 835–841. https://doi.org/10.1097/00042728-200209000-00005

- Gentile, P., Garcovich, S., Bielli, A., Scioli, M. G., Orlandi, A., & Cervelli, V. (2017). The Effect of Platelet-Rich Plasma in Hair Regrowth: A Randomized Placebo-Controlled Trial. Stem Cells Translational Medicine, 6(4), 1016–1023. https://doi.org/10.5966/sctm.2016-0257

- Gupta, A. K., & Foley, K. A. (2019). Platelet-rich plasma for androgenetic alopecia: A review of the literature and proposed treatment protocol. Journal of Dermatological Treatment, 30(5), 396–399. https://doi.org/10.1080/09546634.2018.1530440

- Dhurat, R., & Chitallia, J. (2015). The evolution of treatments for androgenetic alopecia: A review of the current and potential therapies. Journal of Cosmetic Dermatology, 14(4), 253–262. https://

doi.org/10.1111/jocd.12155

- Almohanna, H. M., Ahmed, A. A., Tsatalis, J. P., & Tosti, A. (2019). The role of vitamins and minerals in hair loss: A review. Dermatology and Therapy, 9(1), 51–70. https://doi.org/10.1007/s13555-018-0278-6

- Trüeb, R. M. (2009). Oxidative stress in ageing of hair. International Journal of Trichology, 1(1), 6–14. https://doi.org/10.4103/0974-7753.51923

- Amaral GP, de Carvalho NR, Barcelos RP, et al. Protective action of ethanolic extract of Rosmarinus officinalis L. in gastric ulcer prevention induced by ethanol in rats. Food Chem Toxicol. 2017;55:48-55. doi:10.1016/j.fct.2012.12.038

- Romeu CR, Botta Ferret E, Díaz Finalé Y. Phytochemical characterization of rosemary (Rosmarinus officinalis L.) essential oil and in vitro evaluation of its acaricidal activity. Fitosanidad. 2007;11(2):75-78.

- Panahi, Y., Taghizadeh, M., Marzony, E. T., & Sahebkar, A. (2015). Rosemary oil vs minoxidil 2% for the treatment of androgenetic alopecia: A randomized comparative trial. Skinmed, 13(1), 15-21.

- Young, H. Y., Luo, Y. L., Cheng, H. Y., Hsieh, W. C., Liao, J. C., & Peng, W. H. (2014). The hair growth-promoting effect of peppermint oil and its efficacy in the C57BL/6 mouse model. Toxicological Research, 30(4), 297–304. https://doi.org/10.5487/TR.2014.30.4.297

- Lee, H. J., & Lee, S. H. (2016). The

effect of lavender oil on hair growth. Journal of Ethnopharmacology, 189, 407-413. https://doi.org/10.1016/j.jep.2016.05.049

- Satchell, A. C., Saurajen, A., Bell, C., & Barnetson, R. S. (2002). Treatment of dandruff with 5% tea tree oil shampoo. Journal of the American Academy of Dermatology, 47(6), 852-855. https://doi.org/10.1067/mjd.2002.122734

- Hay, I. C., Jamieson, M., & Ormerod, A. D. (1998). Randomized trial of aromatherapy: Successful treatment for alopecia areata. Archives of Dermatology, 134(11), 1349–1352. https://doi.org/10.1001/archderm.134.11.1349

- Cho, Y. H., Lee, S. Y., Jeong, D. W., Lee, S. J., Kim, E. S., & Lee, J. G. (2014). Effect of pumpkin seed oil on hair growth in men with androgenetic alopecia: A randomized, double-blind, placebo-controlled trial. Evidence-Based Complementary and Alternative Medicine, 2014, 1–6. https://doi.org/10.1155/2014/549721

- Todorov, G., Mihaylova, N., & Kapchina-Toteva, V. (2014). Castor bean (Ricinus communis L.) – A review of its potential in the treatment of hair loss. International Journal of Pharmacognosy and Phytochemical Research, 6(3), 485–489.

- Langan, S. M., & Patel, P. (2019). The role of iron in hair loss: A systematic review. Dermatology and Therapy, 32(5), 827-838. https://doi.org/10.1111/dth.12789

- Fabbrocini, G., Cantelli, M., & Tosti, A. (2021). Nutritional supplements in the treatment of hair loss. Dermatology and Therapy, 34(4), 1-12. https://doi.org/10.1111/dth.14919

- Duan, X., Yang, Z., & Zhang, Z. (2014). Omega-3 fatty acids and their potential role in hair loss prevention. Journal of Dermatological Treatment, 25(5), 395-402. https://doi.org/10.3109/09546634.2013.842168

- Zahed, F., & Naderi, N. (2020). The impact of antioxidants on hair health: A systematic review. Journal of Cosmetic Dermatology, 19(5), 1122-1131. https://doi.org/10.1111/jocd.13205

- Sinclair, R. D. (2016). Hair loss in men and women: The role of nutrition. Journal of Dermatology, 43(3), 341-348. https://doi.org/10.1111/1346-8138.13343

- Pichardo, L., García, P., & Pérez, S. (2017). Vitamins and trace elements in the management of hair loss. Dermatologic Therapy, 30(3), 1-10. https://doi.org/10.1111/dth.12678

- Hoffman, J. R., & Falvo, M. J. (2021). Protein intake and hair growth: Understanding the relationship. International Journal of Sports Nutrition and Exercise Metabolism, 31(2), 98-103. https://doi.org/10.1123/ijsnem.2020-0300

- Hosseini, S. A., & Ghaffari, H. (2020). The role of zinc and selenium in hair health: Review of clinical evidence. Journal of Clinical & Aesthetic Dermatology, 13(4), 21-29.

- Avci, P., Gupta, A., Sadasivam, M., Vecchio, D., Pam, Z., Pam, N., & Hamblin, M. R. (2014). Low-level laser (light) therapy (LLLT) in skin: stimulating, healing, restoring. Seminars in Cutaneous Medicine and Surgery, 33(4), 283–290. https://doi.org/10.12788/j.sder.0099

- Lanzafame, R. J., Blanche, R. R., Bodian, A. B., Chiacchierini, R. P., Fernandez-Obregon, A., & Kazmirek, E. R. (2013). The growth of human scalp hair mediated by visible red light laser and LED sources in males. Lasers in Surgery and Medicine, 45(8), 487–495. https://doi.org/10.1002/lsm.22173

- Leavitt, M., Charles, G., Heyman, E., Michaels, D., & Waldman, A. (2009). HairMax LaserComb laser phototherapy device in the treatment of male androgenetic alopecia: a randomized, double-blind, sham device-controlled, multicentre trial. Clinical Drug Investigation, 29(5), 283–292. https://doi.org/10.2165/00044011-200929050-00001

- Egorov, E. A., Akhmadeev, N. A., & Kirillova, T. A. (2020). Effectiveness of low-level laser therapy for androgenetic alopecia: A systematic review and meta-analysis. Journal of Cosmetic Dermatology, 19(12), 3221–3231. https://doi.org/10.1111/jocd.13806

- Kim, H. H., Yoon, J., Park, H. Y., & Cho, A. R. (2013). Evaluation of hair regrowth after low-level laser therapy using standardized macrophotography and phototrichogram analysis. International Journal of Trichology, 5(4), 193–197. https://doi.org/10.4103/0974-7753.125605

- Dhurat, R., Sukesh, M. S., Avhad, G., Dandale, A., Pal, A., & Pund, P. (2013). Randomized evaluator-blinded study of effect of microneedling in androgenetic alopecia: A pilot study. International Journal of Trichology, 5(1), 6–11. https://doi.org/10.4103/0974-7753.114700

- Faghihi, G., Iraji, F., & Maleki, M. (2020). Microneedling combined with topical minoxidil in the treatment of androgenetic alopecia: A systematic review. Journal of Cosmetic Dermatology, 19(2), 271–276. https://doi.org/10.1111/jocd.13147

- Garcia, A., & Thibaut, S. (2021). "Stress and Hair Loss: A Systematic Review" - International Journal of Trichology.

Pascoe, M., et al. (2017). "The Impact of Meditation on Cortisol and Inflammatory Markers: A Meta-Analysis" - Psychoneuroendocrinology.

- Leung, L., & Davis, A. (2018). "Endorphin Release and Physical Activity: Mechanisms and Implications" - Journal of the American College of Cardiology.

- Irish, L. A., et al. (2015). "Sleep Quality and Hair Health: The Role of Cortisol in Hair Growth" - Sleep Medicine Reviews.

- Caccamese, A., et al. (2020). "Yoga and its Impact on Mental and Physical Health" - Complementary Therapies in Medicine.

- Sato, Y., & Ueda, T. (2016). Scalp massage for improving hair density and growth: A randomized controlled trial. Eplasty, 16, e18.

- Choi, S. Y., & Kim, S. S. (2019). Effects of scalp massage on hair regrowth and hair follicle density in alopecia areata: A prospective, randomized controlled study. Journal of Dermatology, 46(11), 1037-1044.

- Lee, W. R., & Lee, J. H. (2013). The effect of scalp massage on hair growth and regeneration in alopecia patients: A pilot study. Dermatologic Surgery, 39(5), 777-784.

- Kim, M. H., Lee, H. K., & Kim, S. Y. (2017). Massage therapy as a complement to hair loss treatments in androgenetic alopecia: A review of evidence. Journal of Korean Medical Science, 32(7), 1082-1091.

- Mirmirani, P., & Shapiro, J. (2016). Shampoo and conditioner ingredients and their impact on scalp health and hair growth. Journal of Dermatological Treatment, 27(4), 370-376.

- Jang, Y. A., & Lee, J. Y. (2015). The role of scalp care in hair growth: A review of clinical and laboratory studies. International Journal of Trichology, 7(2), 78-84.

Thank you so much for making it to the end of this book!

I deeply appreciate the time you took to read my work. As an independent author, your support means the world to me. My goal is to provide valuable insights and make a positive difference in your health and well-being.

If you have a moment, just 60 seconds, leaving an honest review on Amazon would mean everything to me. Your feedback not only helps me grow but also guides others who might benefit from this book.

To leave your feedback:

1.- Open your camera app
2.- Point your mobile device at the QR code below
3.- The review page will appear in your web browser

Or
Check for "Hair Growth Treatment" in Amazon

I love hearing about your experience with it, your feedback is invaluable!

Check out my other books here:

You can also join my Telegram community
to discover new releases and more:

Thank you once again for your support!